The Amazing Effects of

Massage Therapy

on

Body Image.

by

Craig Botha

The Amazing Effects of Massage Therapy on Body Image.

By Craig Botha
craig@medicalmassage.co.za

ISBN: 154074485X
ISBN-13: 978-1540744852

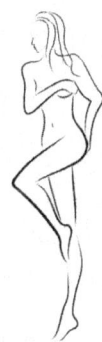

Table of Contents

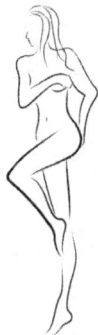

Introduction

Everybody wants to feel and look good, but what does that mean. Most men know that it's like a trap when his wife asks asks "Do I look good in this dress?" or "Do these pants make my bum look fat?" Women (and to an increasing extent, men as well) are concerned about their body image. Most men and women have a healthy view of their own bodies, and see themselves as they really are, and enjoy their bodies. There are however a number of people who have a distorted view of what they look like, an unhealthy body image. Even people who have a realistic view of their own bodies, struggle to enjoy life fully, because they are embarrassed about their bodies, and I would also call this an unhealthy body image. A lot of reading research, and personal experience has lead me to believe that massage can help heal a persons body image.

For over 10 years I have practised as a therapeutic massage therapist. Most of my work is sports massage related, but not all of it. Many of my patients have all different kinds of medical conditions, and different forms of stress. However, a number of my patients have noted that the massage has helped them to feel a lot better about themselves on a psychological level as well, particularly with regard to body image. They feel much more confident in themselves, and a lot more positive about life in general.

This prompted me to do some research, both from an academic point of view and from a practical point of view. I started by trying to find out if any other people had researched this aspect of massage. Some have, but the studies were very small. I also tried to find out what factors contribute to a poor body image, because that could possibly explain why massage could be effective at improving body image. After that, I decided to embark on a practical research program to find out if massage is actually able to help to improve body image, what the mechanisms behind this phenomenon are, if it works for all women, if not why not? Oh, and also I hoped to quantify it. This practical part of the research involved massaging a large group of women a number of times to see if this improved their body image at all.

In my research I only looked at the effects of massage on body image in women. Being a man myself, I expect that the results could be even more amazing when men receive a regular massage, because I believe men are more physical beings, and respond to touch in a more powerful way.

So, like any good research project does, I started with a question:

Can therapeutic massage be used as a treatment to improve a person's body image?

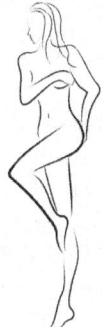

Chapter 1

What is body image anyway?

This is a simple question, but the answer is not as straight forward as one might hope. You might think "what a silly question, body-image is obviously..." The thing is, that body-image means different things to different people. It took me a while to realise this, and I only really found this out half way through my research with real people.

For some women, body-image means a person's perception of what their body looks like. For instance, some people see themselves differently to what they really look like; they might view themselves as very fat, when in fact they are not. Instead, a person with a healthy body-image sees their own body as it really is, whether it be fat or thin, or tall or short or pretty, or what ever the case is.

For other people, body image means "how a person feels in their own body". This view says that a person with a healthy body-image will enjoy their body and feel comfortable in it, no matter what they look like. Therefore, people with a healthy body-image can feel happy and confident and enjoy physical things in their own body, regardless of what they look like, while people with a poor body-image can't enjoy their bodies, even if they believe that they have a fantastic looking body.

I discovered that there are also people who have the view that body image is all about the way clothes look on them. This was a surprise to me, and fascinated me. One of the women in my study group said that she had a fantastic body-image, because she felt that she looks very good in her clothes. I found this very odd, because if we break this down, your body image relies on your clothing budget, and that is the beginning and the end of it. Such a person only needs to be able to afford clothes that look good on her, and she is happy. If this is your understanding of body image, then I feel a bit sorry for you if you don't have a big clothing budget, because you're never going to have the best clothes, and therefore, you can't possibly have a good body-image. I obviously have a problem with that understanding of body image, and don't think it is a healthy one. However, I have given quite a bit of thought to this one, and I think that there is a small grain of truth to this, because if you have a healthy body-image, you are automatically going to feel good in the clothes that you wear. Yes, I have come to believe that a person with a healthy body-image, will feel good about their bodies no matter what clothes they are wearing. Conversely, if you have a poor body image, you may feel that your clothes make you look fat, even if they don't.

Lastly, there are those people who hold to the view that body-image is all about how you feel in the nude. According to this view, you have a healthy body-image if you can get naked and feel comfortable, and a person with a poor body-image will be totally uncomfortable naked, even in front of their own husband or wife, or even when they are alone. I believe this to be partly true. Only partly true though, because culture plays a huge role in this, as we will see later on.

My own view is that all of these views of body image contribute to a proper understanding of what body image really is.

Dictionary definition of body image

If we look up body image in a dictionary, we might find something like the following:

bod·y im·age
noun: body image; plural noun: body images.
The subjective picture or mental image of one's own body.

Web search results for a definition of body image:

What is body image?

In this part of my research I decided to try and find out what a Google search would reveal when I asked it what body image is. Many of the results were interesting and I have presented them here for you.

www.nationaleatingdisorders.org describes body image in the following way:
Body image is how you see yourself when you look in the mirror or when you picture yourself in your mind. It encompasses:
What you believe about your own appearance (including your memories, assumptions, and generalizations).

- How you feel about your body, including your height, shape, and weight.
- How you sense and control your body as you move.
- How you feel in your body, not just about your body.

Negative Body Image:
- A distorted perception of your shape: you perceive parts of your body unlike they really are.

- You are convinced that only other people are attractive and that your body size or shape is a sign of personal failure.
- You feel ashamed, self-conscious, and anxious about your body.
- You feel uncomfortable and awkward in your body.

Positive Body Image:
- A clear, true perception of your shape: you see the various parts of your body as they really are.
- You celebrate and appreciate your natural body shape and you understand that a person's physical appearance says very little about their character and value as a person.
- You feel proud and accepting of your unique body and refuse to spend an unreasonable amount of time worrying about food, weight, and calories.
- You feel comfortable and confident in your body.[1]

au.reachout.com describes body image in this way:

Body image is your attitude towards your body - how you see yourself, how you think and feel about the way you look and how you think others perceive you. Your body image can be influenced by your own beliefs and attitudes as well as those of society, the media and peer groups.

An unhealthy body image is thinking your body is disgusting, unsightly or not good enough. For example, thinking that you look too fat even thought others tell you this is not true, thinking that you're not pretty enough or muscular enough. It can also mean believing what you look like determines your value as a person. Someone with negative body image can become fixated on trying to change their actual body shape.

---

[1] https://www.nationaleatingdisorders.org/what-body-image

A healthy body image is being comfortable in your own skin, being happy most of the time with the way you look, and feeling good with yourself. It's about valuing who you are not what you look like.[2]

The four aspects of body image:

nedc.com.au has the view that there are four aspects to body image and present it in this way:

How you see your body is your perceptual body image. This is not always a correct representation of how you actually look. For example, a person may perceive themselves as overweight when they are actually underweight.

The way you feel about your body is your affective body image. This relates to the amount of satisfaction or dissatisfaction you feel about your shape, weight and individual body parts.

The way you think about your body is your cognitive body image. This can lead to preoccupation with body shape and weight. For example, some people believe they will feel better about themselves if they are thinner or more muscular.

Behaviours in which you engage as a result of your body image encompass your behavioural body image. When a person is dissatisfied with the way they look, they may isolate themselves because they feel bad about their appearance or employ destructive behaviours (e.g. excessive exercising, disordered eating) as a means to change appearance.[3]

Brown University describe body image like this:
Body image includes:

- How we perceive our bodies visually.
- How we feel about our physical appearance; how we think and talk to ourselves about our bodies.
- Our sense of how other people view our bodies.
- Our sense of our bodies in physical space (kinesthetic perception).

---

2   http://au.reachout.com/what-is-body-image
3   http://www.nedc.com.au/body-image

- Our level of connectedness to our bodies.[4]

So, we can see that universities have quite a bit to say on the internet about body image, and that it is quite complex, involving aspects such as what we believe we look like, how we feel, how we believe others see us, how this affects our behaviour, and that there can be factors outside of us that influence our body image. Factors such as society, pear group, culture etc.

---

4   https://www.brown.edu/Student_Services/Health_Services/Health_Education/nutrition_&_eating_concerns/body_image.php

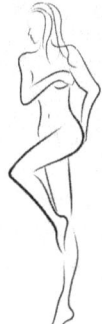

Chapter 2

Psychology of body image

By now we see, that not everybody has a healthy body image, and that many people have a distorted or unhealthy body image that prevents them from enjoying life to the full, and may even handicap them. One question that comes to mind is "how did those of us who struggle with our body image get to this point?" or "What happened in our personal development that might have had an effect on how we see ourselves?"

There are a number of causes that result in poor, or distorted body image. According to Greene and Goodrich-Dunn, some of these causes include the following:

- Abuse - Abuse can result in poor self-esteem, which can lead to a lack of close and trusting relationships or to body image issues (particularly sexual abuse victims), which in turn can result in eating disorders (2013:247).
- Culture/media - Fat, body shape, body image, and fat's connection to health are obsessions in Western culture, particularly for women (2013:256).
- Anorexia - "A person with anorexia usually has body image disturbances, which means that the person perceives (not just believes) that they are fat" (2013:254).
- Sexual Addiction - "... the sex addict can feel sensation that is not sexual as sexualized and thereby begins to "fill in" his body... Due to this fixation, they commonly feel bad about their body image, which is based on how they interpret images of their body" (2013:253).
- PTSD – Post Traumatic Stress Disorder may result in "body memories"... suicidal thoughts over Body Image distortions; dissociative experiences (disconnection between mind and body, not being in one's body) (2013:246). These could be experiences such as the loss of a body part in an accident, or from illness such as cancer, particularly breast cancer, or other traumatic experiences.
- There are many traumatic experiences that can lead to dissociation. This dissociation can be very extreme, and in the extreme there are different dissociative disorders, including:
- Amnesia.
- Depersonalisation Disorder (feeling detached form your body, or that your body is not real).
- Dissociative Fugue (fugue is a kind of mind travel which can last for days).
- Dissociative Identity Disorder (DID), which is a type of multiple personality disorder. [5]

---

5   http://www.mind.org.uk/information-support/types-of-mental-health-problems/dissociative-disorders/#.U3nic4bChMU

Other authors site some other causes for distorted body image: Sinclair (2005:23-25) describes the affect that parenting can have on a child during different stages of childhood, and how this can affect our body image.

- Infancy – Touch is the most mature and developed of all the senses at birth, so touch is very important in the development of a child's body image during infancy. "The construction of body image begins in the first few days of life... during this period somatosensory (bodily sensations) stimulation and tactile stimulation, in particular are critical for developing a healthy body image. Rocking, holding and **massaging** are excellent ways to meet the need...When infants lack adequate sensory stimulation, especially that of touch and movement, their body image as children will be weak and possibly distorted... They will be anxious and have difficulty forming normal emotional attachments to significant others and their ego development will be impaired... Eating disorders may be an attempt to self-cure such early touch deprivation. At the other extreme... Physical or sexual abuse can weaken the sense of body being whole..The invasiveness and use of physical restraint in some medical procedures can also affect body image. The result may be that the child has a weak sense of her body as a private domain" (2005:23-24).

- Middle Childhood – At ages 6-12, children begin to compare their bodies with those around them...Cultural attitudes begin to influence the child's body image. Eg. a fat child in a culture where it is viewed as healthy, will be treated differently in a society where thinness equals beauty. If they have been teased because they look different, children who are disabled may see their bodies as ugly or deformed. Childhood teasing about appearance leads to negative body image and a tendency to develop an eating disorder (2005:24).

- Adolescence - The onset of adolescence confronts all children with the task of revisiting their body image... to accommodate the many normal changes in body structure that occur. Teenagers are more self-conscious and increasingly preoccupied with their body image, asking "am I normal". This is accompanied with frequent comparison of his or her own body with those of other teenagers (and with those in the media who are perceived as perfect), and increased interest in sexual anatomy and physiology. Dieting, exercise, and cosmetic surgery such as liposuction, and breast enhancement surgery, are becoming increasingly common in teenage girls (In the USA), and may be used to help make the body fit the cultural ideals. Women with mothers who were critical of their appearance are more likely to have a negative body image. (2005:24).

Culture and religion:

The society that we grow up in is bound to have an influence on how we develop as people, and body image is no exception. Our culture will teach us how to present our bodies, what makes for a beautiful body, and what makes for an ugly body.

Philip J. Lee writes, "Gnostics of all eras have ··· maintained a most profound mistrust of the body, regarding it as the enemy without that constantly tries to undo the best efforts of the soul within" (1987:130). This kind of gnostic view has filtered into Christian/western culture for centuries, since the beginning of Christianity, even though it is not a Biblical view. The result is a body/mind detachment.

Christians and Christian cultures tend to compartmentalise these areas of body, spirit and mind too much.

Mrs. Knaster is a leading personality in the world of massage in Americaland.. She has edited massage journals, written a number of books, and been involved in a huge amount of research. She interviewed a number of religious leaders for her research. One of the pastors that she interviewed said:

"We become disconnected and dysfunctional." (2000:nn)

We keep the spiritual part of us locked up and bring it out for church. We hide the physical part of ourselves while at church, because it is just way too worldly and unspiritual (Gnostic Influence). Sometimes we feel that we need to leave our intellect at the door when we go to church, because we think it should be kept separate from faith. This is in spite of the fact that Jesus teaches a holistic message, and Himself, being perfect, had a human body.

Another way in which culture or religion can affect body image, is if a person's cult or faith are not mainstream for the area that they live in. This can drastically reduce the size of the pool of potential marriage partners. If such a person finds it difficult to find a soul mate/life partner in that community, it can lead to a sense of inadequacy, which can affect self-confidence, self-image, and in turn body image.

Neglect:

We often think of abuse as being limited to physical, emotional, and sexual. However, Childline South Africa list another form of abuse as 'Neglect'[6]. Neglect can include: a lack of supervision, protection, adequate clothing, medical and dental care, education opportunities, proper hygiene or emotional support. If a child is deprived of any one of these things, it could lead to a sense of inadequacy, which in turn, can affect body image.

---

6 http://www.childlinesa.org.za/index.php/documents-for-download/doc_download/197-recognising-childabuse

Psychology of body image

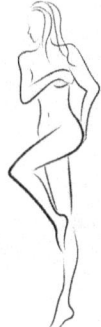

Chapter 3

The psychology of touch

We have seen in the previous chapter that touch deprivation, and inappropriate touch (sexual abuse or physical abuse) can have destructive effects on the development of a persons psychology and specifically on body-image. The reverse is also true, that touch and massage can be extremely therapeutic and helpful in the treatment of patients who have a poor body image and other psychological problems as a result of touch deprivation, or abuse, even emotional abuse.

It is no accident that Gary Chapman (2007) includes physical touch as one of the five love languages in his popular book *The Five Love Languages*. According to Gary Chapman, touch is one of five ways that we understand love when it is communicated to us, and it is one of the five ways we communicate love to others. There are some difficulties that need to be negotiated though. These difficulties are negative responses to touch, so let us have a look at some of them.

Touch can trigger buried memories (Sinclare 2013:160) - Sometimes these memories can can be good memories, but often these memories can be quire bad, even traumatic memories.

The patient will associate the emotions that accompany those memories with the massage therapist. This can either result in an inappropriate attachment to and affection for the therapist, or unwarranted mistrust, discomfort, or even animosity towards the massage therapist.

Sandy Fritz writes:

"Often only pieces of memory are retrieved. This is common with body memories. The massage may trigger a physiologic response, yet no visual or sequential memory is retrievable. Just because a person does not remember who, what, when why, or how does not mean that the memory is not valid" (2010:nn).

In a chapter on spontaneous recall of abuse memories, Renee Fredrickson writes "A triggering event or catalyst starts the memories flowing. The survivor then experiences the memories as a barrage of images about the abuse and related details." Ferdrickson advocates massage therapy as a method of retrieving repressed memories. She writes: "Massage therapy or body manipulation techniques access body memories for survivors. As certain places on the body are touched or certain movements are made, memories of abuse may surfaced... Body work is often used by survivors to aid in memory work" (1992:98). Of course, sexual abuse is not the only physical memory a person can have triggered by massage.

Not only can massage trigger memories, but it can trigger emotional release. Patients may be going through an emotionally stressful time, or recently have gone through such a period of emotional stress. An example might be when somebody goes through a divorce, and all the stress that goes with that. Because massage works on an autonomic level to create a parasympathetic nervous response it has a physiological affect on the endocrine system. This in turn can trigger an emotional release. This can be very confusing for the patient. This is summed up in the words of one of my clients "Why do I feel like crying??? But I want more???"

It is important to continue treatment sessions through these awkward and uncomfortable periods for reframing to take place. Reframing is a process of psychological change. There are a number of techniques that psychotherapists use to enable patients to reframe certain psychologies. In the case of body image, I believe massage to be one very powerful way to facilitate reframing.

The psychology of touch

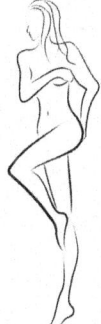

Chapter 4

Massage your body image better

In this chapter I want to do some academic research into the way massage can help us to heal or at least improve our body image. I'm the first to admit that body image is complex and that healing would also be complex. As a result, massage is not the only therapy. I believe that massage is a vital part of of the healing process, but that for somebody really struggling with poor, or even self destructive body image problems, that they do need to be in the care of a psychologist and that massage should only be one of a combination of therapies to be employed for healing. That said, I believe it to be a very important therapy.

The role of massage.

Fritz writes: "Because massage produces changes in the nervous and endocrine systems and is a source of sensory stimulation, a state that holds a memory pattern for a client could be recreated. This may help a person resolve and integrate a past experience..." (2010:nn).

Although there is a lot of literature available on the effectiveness of massage in restoring a healthy body image. There is not much literature available which describes the role of massage in restoring a healthy body image, or the mechanisms behind it's effectiveness. Sinclare writes the most on the subject. However most of her research is centred on child development. She does write one sentence that could hold the key to the mechanism for it working in adults though. She writes:

> **"Massage is physically pleasurable and leaves a strong impression in the child's mind, because pleasurable touch enhances the perception of the touched part"** (2013:25).

A positive body image accepts the body and respects it by attending to its needs and engaging in healthy behaviours. In a qualitative study, many college women with a positive body image indicated that they regularly received massages to take care of, appreciate, and pamper their body, showing that they view massage as pleasurable. Massage treatment could function as a positive feedback cycle, by not only lessening negative feelings about the body through increasing body acceptance, but also by associating emergent positive feelings with the body and partaking in a behaviour that honours and relaxes the body. Massage could also improve body image by reducing women's objectification of their bodies. A woman with a negative body image often views her body as an object to be evaluated. Women in western cultures learn to survey their bodies through the eyes of their culture to avoid negative judgement. A woman can feel that her body brings unhappiness and shame because it is perceived as not measuring up to society's ideals. A woman who receives a massage, can let her body become a vehicle for the experience of pleasure. Women who hold a negative body image may avoid massage due to shame or embarrassment.[7] Even though it is the very thing that will bring healing and dispel the shame and embarrassment. Although I searched quite a lot, I didn't find many practical studies done to establish the effectiveness of massage in improving body image. In fact, I only found two studies. The first study I found is the study conducted by scientists from Bridgewater State University, MA, USA looked at the effect of massage on state body image.

In the study conducted by the Bridgewater University, they recruited forty-nine female university students; they were randomly assigned to either a massage condition (given a massage) or a control condition (given a lecture of some kind to improve body image). It was hypothesized that participants in the massage condition would report an improved state of body image following the intervention when compared to participants in the control condition. As predicted, participants in the massage condition reported a more favourable state body image than participants in the control condition post-manipulation (after the massage). Certain body image evaluations were moderately associated with views that massage is pleasurable, with the link between Body Areas Satisfaction and viewing massage as pleasurable reaching significance.

In this study, it is conclusive that the female university students reported feeling better about themselves and their bodies after having received a massage. Meanwhile the control group, who did not receive any massage, showed no change in their attitudes. A woman's negative view of her body can make the body seem untouchable and grotesque. Massage can be a vehicle to have a positive experience in the the body, and could potentially break through these negative body image attitudes. Nevertheless, a woman who holds negative thoughts about her body may be less apt to seek out massage therapy. This attitude will need to be addressed for massage to be a viable therapeutic option. In addition to relaxation and a shift in focus from the body as an

---

7   http://true.massage-research.com/2013/06/massage-and-body-image.html

object, regular massage could help change negative thoughts about the body as the body becomes associated with the good feelings that it brings through the massage experience.[8]

This study at Bridgewater State University done as an investigation into the link between massage and body image, was done by Bonnie Fletcher, but It was a very limited research. The research of 23 university girls, which is a good size group, But only half were massaged, making it a group of 11 or 12 that were actually massaged. This is a very small group. The other half of the were just a control group. No details are given about the style or modality of the massage, or even the extent of the massage. The only detail given about the massage is that the women first indicated on a diagram, which body parts they did not want to be touched. The research did indicate that massage does indeed affect body image positively, but gives no reasons why it should work. (Fletcher 2009).

The second study into massage and body image that I could find was an even smaller study, it was a study on one person, which is statistically pointless as far as I am concerned.

In 2012 Maxfield and Holland conducted a research study on the effect of massage on body image. Although the research consisted of weekly massage sessions over 4 weeks, it only had one massage subject (one person, a dancer). She did have an improved body image. Not much can be learned from this study. The type of massage used was Swedish massage, and was limited to what ever area the patient felt needed working on, on that particular day. (Maxfield and Holland. 2012).

So with such an underwhelming amount of actual studies that I could find, I felt that I needed to find out the answers myself. This is when I decided to conduct my own study, on as large a group of women as I could possibly find. I felt that the study needed to be both statistically significant in terms of the number of women, and in terms of the number of massages given. I also thought that it would be important to be specific about the kind of massage that I was going to do. So, let me first look at what massage is all about. In particular I want to define what therapeutic massage is.

---

8   true.massage-research.com/2013/06/massage-and-body-image.html

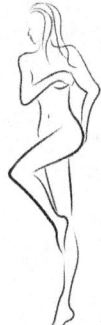

Chapter5

What is a therapeutic massage therapist?

Now that I had decided to do my own study on how well massage can improve body image. I thought that it would be important to actually first try and define what massage is (if that is possible) and then to choose   particular type of massage and run with that, in order to get consistent results that could be reliable.

You may be surprised at how often I get asked the simple question "What is massage therapy?" It's a question I get asked regularly, and I am still surprised each time I am asked. I'm surprised because it is probably the oldest therapy known to mankind. If I bump myself against the table as I walk past, I stop and rub the pain away, or try to at any rate. It's a natural response, it works. That is the most basic form of massage therapy.

In South Africa, the massage therapy profession is legislated in the Allied Health Professions Act, and all of its associated regulations. In one such regulation, "Therapeutic Massage Therapy" is defined as "...a massage therapy treatment delivered for a specific therapeutic outcome."[9] 'Massage', in relation to massage therapy, means "...the mobilisation of soft tissue."[10] So a Therapeutic Massage Therapist is an Allied Health Professional who uses massage (physical manipulation of soft tissue) as a therapeutic intervention for many physical, medical, and stress related conditions.

Scope of Practice of Massage Therapy

According to the Massage Therapy Association of South Africa, the scope of practice is defined as:

> "Verbal and physical **assessment** and evaluation of a patient's condition for the purpose of evaluating the state of health and the delivery of a treatment regime to meet the needs of the patient....
>
> **Application** of therapeutic massage therapy treatments by the use of hands with reference to the treatment and prevention of conditions of illness in any patients. These are facilitated by:
>
> Therapeutic **massage techniques** i.e. the manual mobilisation of soft tissue structures" (MTASA:nn)[11].

Definition of Massage Therapy

Massage is very difficult to define, even if people are clear in their understanding of what massage is. Massage, according to Akhoury Sinha's, definition is "any technique, be it manual or mechanical, which imparts mechanical energy to the soft tissue of body though the skin... in order to elicit certain physiological or psychological effect which can be utilised for therapeutic,

---

9   Allied Health Professions of South Africa Regulation 127 (2001:6)
10   Allied Health Professions of South Africa Regulation 127 (2001:5)
11   Massage Therapy Assosiation of South Africa https://mtasa.co.za/about-mta/scope-of-practice/

restorative or preventative purposes either on a sick or a healthy individual..." (2001:2).

The US Department Of Labor (yes that is how Americans spell labour), defines massage as follows: "Massage therapists treat clients by using touch to manipulate the soft-tissue muscles of the body. With their touch, therapists relieve pain, help rehabilitate injuries, improve circulation, relieve stress, increase relaxation, and aid in the general wellness of clients." [12]

There are a variety of different massage modalities. Most massage modalities involve the use of therapeutic oils massaged into an affected area of the body, or even the whole body, as in the case of a full body massage. Massage has been part of every major culture since the beginning of time, and as a result, there are many types of massage. We call these different types of massage *modalities*. Swedish massage is one such modality, and is the traditional Western style of massage. Virginia Cowen (2011:96) describes Swedish massage as the most common form of western massage, based on an understanding of anatomy and physiology and is performed using a series of massage stroke sequences aimed to affect different tissues of the body, using oils or other lubricants .

According to Calvert (who has written a fantastic book on the history of massage) wrote "A proper definition of massage must include not only its therapeutic role and historic development, but also its capacity to nurture and support - to feed the spirit, bind relationships, and please the senses. Massage is about relationships and it's about healing. **Massage is the highest order of touch**" (2002:11).

A Short History of Massage

The word massage has not always been used to describe this type of treatment. In fact, the word *massage* is a very new English word. However the practice has an ancient history in most cultures. Calvert (2002:1) describes the history of massage as going back thousands of years in Egypt, China, Greece, Hawaii and Australia.

---

12   United States Department of Labor, http://www.bls.gov/ooh/healthcare/massage-therapists.htm

Hippocrates, widely considered the father of modern medicine, described many treatments involving massage, though he used the terms rubbing, or stroking.

In a study of healing in Biblical times, Pieter Craffert (1999:1-144) describes three types of people who would call themselves doctors: There was the type that would cast spells (what we would call a witch doctor today). There was the type that would practice a mix of natural remedies and massage following the example of Hippocrates, and there was the philosopher type who would really just talk about the disease, being more interested discussing in the prognoses than actually treating the disease.

If we look at the type of medicine that Hippocrates practised, we find that it is not that different to the holistic massage therapist of today. Hippocates believed that massage was a valuable therapeutic tool, he just used the word *anatripsis*, a Greek word related to rubbing (Clavert 2002:44). Hippocrates is quoted as saying "The physician must be experienced in many things, but most assuredly also in rubbing" (Hippocrates, ny:vol vi:100).

The Biblical practice of anointing also has it's origins in massage. Calvert (2002:47) suggests that anointing (a Latin derived word) with oil in the ancient world was in fact massage. Anointing was done throughout history, usually after bathing and served as a skin moisturiser when oil was rubbed onto the skin. In Egypt anointing was believed to afford curative benefits. The favoured oil being a blend of olive oil myrrh, cinnamon, cain, or cassia. Thus the Egyptian practice of anointing of ancient times would have been something we would recognise as massage or aromatherapy today. Incidentally, the difference between massage and aromatherapy is not immediately apparent. Essentially, massage therapy uses oils (which can be therapeutic) to assist in lubrication, while aromatherapy uses massage to apply therapeutic oils to the body.

According to Strong (2011:H4886), the Hebrew for anoint is *mâshach*, a primitive root, to rub with oil. And according to Calvert (2002:2), the Arabic word for massage is '*mass-h*' from the Arabic verb '*mass*', which means 'to touch'. You can see that those two words are very similar.

The Greek words for anoint and anointed are similar in meaning. There are many Greek words in the New Testament of the Bible which are translated as anoint. However word *egchrio* in Revelation 3:18 which is translated as anoint, is derived from the root word *chrio* which means 'to rub with oil' (Strong 2011:G1472). Likewise, the Greek word for one who is anointed is *Christos* which means one who is rubbed with oil (Strong 2011:G5548). This is the word we translate as 'Christ'. Although historically, anointing represents something more symbolic of a massage with oil. This makes a lot of sense if we conceder the intimacy of a massage, and the Egyptian origins of anointing, and anointing as something that happened after a bath to nourish the skin and heal the body, preparing it for a day in the sun. Symbolic anointing may indicate that the one being anointed is clean, washed accepted, and prepared for some task, or to indicate that the one being anointed has the desire for healing.

Yes, this might appear to be a Bible study, but the I believe that symbolic anointing or religious anointing has it's roots in real massage, and represents acceptance. This, is central to understanding why massage can be so effective in improving self confidence and body image.

Holland and Anderson (2011:12) write that massage in Europe died out almost entirely during the Middle Ages, apart from a few dedicated monks in monitories who practice healing techniques.

In their brief section on the history of massage, Holey and Cook (2011:5) give an account of the development of massage. Their account states that many ancient civilisations developed systems of massage. These civilisations included China, India, Arabia, Greece, Italy and Egypt. Massage was used for various medical conditions. The re-emergence of massage in the West is attributed to French missionaries. These missionaries returning from China in the early nineteenth century, brought with them medical writings dating back to 2700BC. These Chinese writings were then translated into French, and this is why some of the terminology still used in massage today is French terminology. Massage for gymnasts was first made popular by Per Henrik Ling of Sweden in 1813. This became known as Swedish massage, which then spread through the West, and institutes for Swedish massage were established in London in 1838 and in New York in 1916. Since then much research and development has happened in Europe and America, resulting in many different modalities of massage.

Synovitz and Larson describe the Lomi lomi Hawaiian massage therapy as being developed by ancient Polynesians and master healers. "The Hawaiian healing philosophy... holds the assumption that everything seeks harmony and love. Massage is related to that philosophy through gently, yet deeply working the muscles with loving hands. It uses continuous long flowing strokes and relaxes the entire being. The therapist may use the forearms as well as the hands so that people who experience it say it feels like gentle waves moving over the body" (2013:185).

The Massage Therapy Association of South Africa (MTASA), formerly known as the Holistic Massage Practitioners Association, was founded in 1989 to work towards the professional recognition of Therapeutic Massage Therapy in South Africa[13]. Massage therapy was only legislated in South Africa in 2001 with an amendment to the Allied Health Professions Act (Act 63 of 1982). This legislation sets minimum standards of training and education, and makes registration with the Allied Health Professions Council of South Africa (a council set up by an act of parliament) compulsory.

---

13   http://www.cosmeticweb.co.za/pebble.asp?relid=681

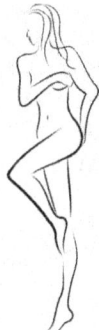

Chapter 6

What is unique about the massage therapy environment?

There are several components of massage therapy that set it apart from an environment where counselling, spiritual direction or psychotherapy might take place. Primary among these are the following:

Dress Code.

Although the therapist is dressed, depending on the extent of the massage, patients are semi-nude, or even totally nude. "Swedish massage is traditionally performed on a massage table with the client unclothed" (Cowen 2011:96). The Hawaiian style of massage with it's long, full body length flowing strokes, is certainly always performed on a patient who is totally naked. This often leads to a relationship of trust, in which the patient feels free to share very personal details of their lives, and often their emotional struggles too. Although this openness might be out of nervousness at first, it certainly develops into a trust relationship with the progresses of time. According to Daniela Aneis, this is one of the reasons why naked yoga is becoming popular. It is "because it helps in re-connecting with other humans in a naked mind-body-and-soul way" (2014:nn).

While it would be highly suspect and unethical for a pastor, counsellor, or psychologist to ask his/her patient to get undressed for a counselling session, massage patients go to a massage therapist for a massage, which by its very nature, involves some level of undress.

Emotional Responses to Physical Touch and Massage.

Touch can bring about emotional healing. In their book *The Psychology of the Body*, Greene and Goodrich-Dun fill over 300 pages on emotional responses to touch, including emotional healing, and emotional release. Often the release of physical and mental stress, triggered by massage, can be accompanied by an emotional release with an outpouring of tears and emotions. Most often this release of emotions has no real explanation other than just a release of tension built up over time. But from time to time that tension has been caused by emotional, physical or even sexual abuse. This is a time when the patient is open to sharing their story, and looking for guidance.

Touch can bring about emotional healing because it is nurturing in the same way that a mother bonds with her new-born child. Greene and Goodrich-Dun (2013:62) warn that a patient can sometimes project negative aspects of their parents onto a massage therapist and respond negatively, even fearfully if that parent was physically or sexually abused. However, if that patient continues with massage therapy, the caring touch can result in psychological re-framing. Touch is then transformed (in the mind and experience of the patient) from something horrible to something enjoyable. However, this does take perseverance and time.

Cheryl Kerrigan, in her book on her own experience of overcoming her eating disorder (ED) writes this about massage:

Lying naked on a table while someone rubs you down is a luxury for most. For me, it's a therapy. Being in tune with and connected to my body is important in my recovery. I must learn to live in this body and accept it, no matter what its size. Lying on the massage table helps me to accomplish that... One would think it would be excruciating for a person with an eating disorder to lie naked and have someone touch the very thing you despise; however, for me it brings me courage, freedom, strength, power, and acceptance. It took time and courage for me to get to that point, but when I was ready to take the risk and push through the fear of exposing myself and my body, the reward was well worth it.

I get naked, lie on the table... take a deep breath and it begins. For ninety minutes I am on that table, my mind and body become one. Sure, for the first seconds ED tries to jump in and tell me that I am so big that all my fat is hanging over the table - but I talk back and tell him he is a jerk and I am not fat at all. I reframe the negative thoughts into positive ones, and before I know it, my mind is in tune with what the therapist is doing. I can honestly say the time I spend on that table brings me a sense of freedom - freedom from my negative body image and negative thoughts.

I lie there and actually feel my body from the inside out. I feel light all over... I do not judge myself. I feel my body to be the instrument and gift it is... and massage therapy helps me see that, helps me feel that being mindful and in tune in both mind and body! When I leave that tranquil space, I am ready to face the world with a sense of power because I know that my mind and body are learning to become one - to become friends" (2010:nn)

Mirka Knaster, who I quoted earlier, from her doctoral research on the interface between Judaism and Buddhism, published an article in Beliefnet[14], in which she quotes from interviews of Christian and Jewish clergy, from a variety of denominations, who have started to incorporate massage into their counselling, occupation, and prayer retreats. Knaster recounts the story of a pastoral counsellor:

She had been "sexually abused felt split off from part of herself, her psychotherapist recommended body therapy. After receiving massages from a graduate of the Baptist Theological Seminary in her city, she realized that the more she got to know herself through the sessions, the more she was able to embrace all of who she is... By befriending her body in massage, the counselor also learned to accept blessing and grace just for being. Grace was no longer an abstract concept, but a concrete experience" (2000:nn).

Knaster also relates the story of a Protestant interim pastor who worked as a massage therapist and often got horrified looks when other pastors found out that he massaged women while they were naked. He says of conservative Christians...

"The body and the spirit are always at war with one another. They are afraid of their bodies and touch of any kind because they have never come to terms with their own sexuality." He sees massage as a way for people to break down that barrier, redeem the body, and praise God for it (2000:nn).

14   http://www.beliefnet.com/Wellness/2000/08/Touching-Spirit.aspx?p=1

In my personal experience, this holds true for conservative people of any faith, and that massage can break those barriers. In the process they can release some bottled up emotions and memories. This is particularly true for those who have experienced some kind of abuse in their past, be it emotional, physical, or sexual.

As a normal counselling session does not involve such close physical contact, the likelihood of surfacing these kinds of emotions through touch is very small, and the counsellor or psychologist may never know the reason for a counsellee's problem. Even if the counsellor does elicit such and emotional response through touch, he may not have the skill set to use therapeutic touch to being healing. This places the massage therapist in a unique space.

Although the emotions and memories that are surfaced through massage can be very helpful in the counselling process, I am not in favour of digging up past memories in the Freudian style of psychotherapy. This only seeks to find something or someone in one's past to blame for everything that is wrong in one's life at the moment. I am in favour of recognising the past, dealing with it and looking forward.

Greene and Goodrich-Dunn (2013:256) quote a study in which women suffering with anorexia, where treated with massage therapy. The study showed that those receiving massage treatment experienced reduced levels of anxiety, stress, and improved body-image.

What is unique about the massage therapy environment?

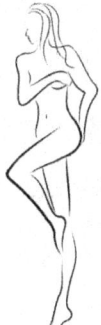

Chapter 7

The Study

The aim of the research study.

I've already said in the introduction that this book is based on the research I did, and that the research question is **Can therapeutic massage be used as a treatment to improve a patient's body image?**

So, what did I set out do do with my research? Well the answer to that is simple: I set out to massage a bunch of women and see if this can result in an improvement in their body image. That way I would know if it actually works or not. In order to do this, I had to find a large enough group of women to massage in order to get some statistical significance. I also had to ask each woman a set of standardised questions before and after massage sessions, so that I could track their progress over the research period, which was five massage sessions for each person (one a week for five weeks).

The massage research modality

Taking into consideration the clients I have who have reported this phenomenon to me: I looked at their treatment records to find out what their treatments had in common. I soon realised that they have all had the same type of massage, namely the Yeru massage.

So, at the outset of this research I decided to find women who would be prepared to come for five full body, Yeru massages, then see what the results are.

The research

Participants were all female. And were really anybody I could find brave enough to take part.

The massage treatment I chose is a modality I developed about 8 years ago which I call a Yeru massage (Yeru being a Hebrew word for 'flow' or 'flowing'. It is a combination of Swedish and Lomi Lomi (Hawaiian) massage, incorporating a lot of full body length rhythmic strokes, which are very good at eliciting an entrainment effect. The massage also includes a lymphatic breast care massage. For this massage to work well practically, the patient needs to be totally naked during the massage.

I chose this type of massage because patients in the past who have commented that they had experienced an improved body image had received this massage. Also, because patients of mine in the past who have experience emotional release of some kind after a massage had all received this massage.

Firstly, the participant (patient) filled in a medical history form and before each massage filled in the following questions:

How comfortable do you feel in your body?
0. 1. 2. 3. 4. 5. 6. 7. 8. 9. 10.

How much do you enjoy your body?
0. 1. 2. 3. 4. 5. 6. 7. 8. 9. 10.

How comfortable are you being naked when you are alone?
0. 1. 2. 3. 4. 5. 6. 7. 8. 9. 10.

How comfortable are you being naked with your partner?
0. 1. 2. 3. 4. 5. 6. 7. 8. 9. 10.

How comfortable are you getting naked for a health exam / beauty treatment etc.?
0. 1. 2. 3. 4. 5. 6. 7. 8. 9. 10.

How would you say your body image affects your life?

I also gave each patient a description of the massage, and asked them to remove as much clothing as they were comfortable with. Some patients were not comfortable removing their underwear, although I still did the full body length strokes. One patient asked for additional draping over the lower private parts as well as the breasts and not to include her breasts in the massage. One patient asked to have her lower private parts to be draped, although she was comfortable being totally naked, she did ask to have her breasts excluded. One patient kept her underwear on and asked not to have her breasts included.

At the end of each session each participant was asked to fill in the following two questions:

7. Would you say that your body image has changed since the treatment started?
0. 1. 2. 3. 4. 5. 6. 7. 8. 9. 10.

8. Any other comments about the treatment?

Mistakes

1. I decided from the beginning to do full body massages, because in the past, it is only women that have had the full body Yeru massage that have reported improved body image. This was a mistake because some women just aren't ready for a full body massage. So, the experience for them is just so horrible that they didn't want to come back for the follow up sessions.

2. Lack of information: I decided from the beginning to give as much information about the massage as I could to prepare each woman for what was to come, but also purposely decided not to give information about possible reactions to the massage. I did this because I wanted the women to experience this for themselves, then tell me about what they felt. This was a mistake, because many were not prepared for the reactions they had or the feelings they experienced, which made them feel totally uncomfortable and didn't want to come back for the follow up sessions.

A reaction that many are not prepared for is sexual arousal. This does not happen to all women. However, It does happen, and it is natural. The problem is not that it happens, but how it is handled. A woman who has not had a full body massage before may not expect to become sexually aroused during the massage. If she does become sexually aroused, and is not ready for it, she may find very difficult to deal with appropriately, and become extremely self concious or have feelings of guilt and decide not to come back. The truth is, that it is a non-even, and as the client returns for more massages, they learn that it is not that big a deal.

The other reaction is triggered memories. If the massage triggers memories that are unpleasant, then she will not want to come back, particularly if she was not warned about them. These triggered memories may be of hurtful experiences in the past.

Triggered emotions, if touch in a certain area of the body triggers an emotion that is unpleasant, then she will not want to come back. (one client in the past described a full body massage as to "touchy feely". The nature of massage is touchy/feely, but if a person is touch deprived, then they may not be able to respond appropriately, and find it overwhelming and unpleasant. This would also be true if their past touch experience has been inappropriate experience such as physical, or sexual abuse.

3. Lack of time: I know from the past ten years that a full body massage takes an hour, so didn't allow for much more time than that for each appointment. This is a mistake, because with the emotions experienced. some patients want to talk, through their feelings, or just take some time to gather themselves. This takes time. So, I need to build time in before the massage for a briefing, and after the massage for a debriefing, besides just the filling in of forms.

I have learned a lot through these mistakes. However, I also lost a number of the volunteers because of these mistakes, and fear that for them, all I have done is reinforce their distorted experience of touch, and their distorted body image.

Lessons learned.

1. Allow for plenty of time before and after the massage, not just for the filling in of forms, but also for briefing and debriefing.
2. Give as much information as possible about the physical massage sequence, and about the possible emotional reactions.
3. The person needs to commit to sticking it out for a number of sessions to get through the awkward stage of negative response to massage, until they start to feel more comfortable.

4. Allow the patient to progress at their own pace with gentle encouragement each session, to take the next step. eg. If the patient is not comfortable with more than just a back massage, then just give a back massage until such time as they are ready (even if apprehensive) to move on. The final goal is to have the patient totally comfortable with a full body that includes breast massage. The big breakthrough does come after the second or third massage like this.

5. It is vitally important that the massage is not sexual i.e. vaginal massage. This non-sexual yet caring touch is what contributes to the re-framing process. I mention this because one patient remarked that the fact that it was full body yet non-sexual, was very liberating and therapeutic.

Other difficulties with research:

There were a number of practical issues that prevented some patients from finishing the course of massage treatments. First is sickness. With the change of the season, a number of patients did get the flu that was going around. Work, and family commitments created difficulties for some people. For some patients completing the five sessions meant chopping and changing appointments, or coming every second week in stead of every week. Some had to abandon the process altogether because of work commitments.

For some it was just too difficult to follow through on the commitment. One woman owns her own business had all the best intentions in the world. She has a very well adjusted body image, enjoys massage, wants to come at least once a month, but doesn't actually have the conviction to carry through on her intentions saying that she is too busy at work, and business comes first.

One patient found the timing didn't work out for her, a mission posting that she has been looking forward to for 3 years finally came through after her second treatment, when it was time for her to move to Angola.

Briefing before the massage.

It is important to sit down with the patient before the first massage and brief them on the extent of the massage, the options that they have, the possible physical or emotional reactions they might experience, as well as the importance of letting me know if I do anything that freaks them out.

The following questions may also help me to determine the extent of what they would be comfortable with for their first massage.

1. Have you had any massages before?
2. Did you enjoy the massages or did you feel uncomfortable?
3. What was the extent of the massages you had in the past? (back, full body).
4. If you felt uncomfortable, in what way did you feel uncomfortable?
5. Were any massages that you had before from a male or female therapist?
6. What are your concerns about the massage you're about to have?
7. What parts of your body would you be totally uncomfortable with me massaging.
8. Are you committed to working through a period of awkwardness that may last for a couple of sessions?

Debriefing after the massage.

It is also important for me to ask two questions after each massage:

1. How do you feel?
2. Will you take note of how you feel in the coming hours and days and let me know before the start of the next massage session?

The second question is because experience tells me that most people have not really had a chance to process their feeling right after the massage, and that it takes a few hours, even a day or two to really get to grips with the experience.

The Study

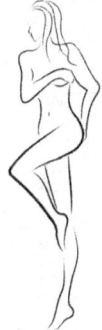

Chapter 8

Research findings

How I collated the results:

This was quite simple. For each massage session, I added up the score for the questions asked before and after the massage session. There were 8 questions with a score out of 10, therefore a score of 80 would be equal to 100% score for good body image. Such a person just doesn't exist. Consistently, it is very easy to track the improvement or deterioration in the woman's body image by seeing how that score increased or decreased. For example if the first score was 30 and the last score was 40, that is an improvement of 10%

Actual results:

I massaged 3 groups of women, for 5 sessions each. Not all the women were able to return for all 5 sessions. Some because of work commitments, etc. I have totally excluded the results from those women who came for only one massage. Before each massage I gave each woman the option of a full body Yeru massage, very few took up that option to start with but by the 5th massage 55% felt comfortable enough to take up that option. Bellow are the results broken up into different groupings:

Overall results: **35.82% improvement.**

Group 1 (5 women):   13.93% improvement.
Group 2 (1 woman):   29.71% improvement.
Group 3 (15 women):   63.81% improvement.

Two women in the 3rd group did have their score go down, one by 9.9% and one by 2.63%.

The following are the results after of the number of massages completed.

Group 1:

After...	Overall improvement
2 massages:	4.34% improvement.
3 massages:	9.44% decrease.
4 massages:	10.23% improvement.
5 massages:	13.93% improvement.

Group 2:

After...	Overall improvement
2 massages:	14% improvement.
3 massages:	22.9% improvement.
4 massages:	28.37% improvement.
5 massages:	29.71% improvement.

Group 3:

After...	Overall improvement
2 massages:	13.12% improvement.
3 massages:	26.36 % improvement.
4 massages:	49.91 % improvement.

5 massages: 63.81% improvement.

The person with the biggest improvement started with a score of 20 and ended with a score of 46 after 5 massages. This is an improvement of 130%.

The person with the highest starting score started on a score of 52 and ended on a score of 59, a 13.46% improvement.

1. Yes, massage does improve body image, even if it is a single massage of a limited part of the body. It is much more effective if it is a full body massage, even more than doubly effective if it is a number of sessions, because the patient becomes much more comfortable with the therapy on follow up treatments. However, a number of full body Yeru massages with the patient totally naked is infinitely more effective, not just at improving body-image, by also at reducing stress, and is still the only massage modality that I have given, that results in a dramatic emotional release.

2. It is when a patient has been informed about what to expect, that a full body, Yeru massage can be extremely effective.

3. The most common reactions to a full body Yeru massage:

•   Emotional release. This may be due to a combination of the relaxing/de-stressing nature of the massage, as well as the liberating experience. But emotional release, feeling very emotional, and even crying are a common response to this massage.

•   Opening up emotionally. In fact, this is even true for many of those who have not graduated to the full body massage, but not every one.

•   Sexual arousal. I found that about 1/3 of the women massaged became sexually aroused. This it totally normal and also totally acceptable. With each subsequent massage, that sexual arousal becomes less significant, and less of an issue for the patient. So, it is vitally important to come for three or four massages after that, to work through the awkward stage and reach a stage where the patient is comfortable. Only two woman responded inappropriately but asking for an erotic massage (this of course, is unacceptable, but still needs to be handled with grace). I found that the risk of this happening is reduced by laying down the ground rules (boundaries) before treatment starts.

- It takes a few sessions of the full body Yeru massage before the patient really feels comfortable, is able to relax, and respond appropriately. It is then that they are really able to enjoy the massage and touch for what it is, a relaxing, caring (even if intimate) touch experience. This is when the patient really starts to feel comfortable in their own body, no matter what their body shape, and they develop a healthy body image. A bonus is that as soon as the patient starts to enjoy their body, they also start to look after it better, and have a more healthy approach to diet and exercise.

4. Almost without exception, women with a poor body image have a lot of hurt in their past, from incidents such as teasing, and verbal abuse to sexual abuse.

5. The level of comfort a woman has with her body seldom has anything to do with what her body actually looks like, but can result in neglect of the body, (lack of exercise, and over eating, or anorexia) which all affect what the body looks like. In other words, given time, a person's body-image may affect what their body looks like, rather than the other way around (their body, affecting their body-image).

6. For what ever reason, some women can be very dishonest about their feelings, i.e. they can tend to fake their comfort level during a massage. This may stem from a willingness to please, and not disappoint the therapist. Asking questions doesn't really gain insight into how comfortable they are with a massage. If they are uncomfortable during a massage they won't tell you. They will even book a second appointment. The time you really find out is when

it is time for them to come for that second appointment and they find an excuse not to come, or they tell you then that they weren't comfortable during the massage.

7. The more information that women have about the massage, e.g. level of undress, body parts included, emotional response, etc. The more comfortable they are during the actual massage.

8. Response from women who don't go totally nude for a massage is rather mixed. Some have said that they feel nurtured. Some just feel totally uncomfortable with the whole massage, even though they didn't go totally nude. Of the women who were brave enough to go totally naked, only one did not feel comfortable enough to return for second massage, and that was because she didn't quite know how to handle the sexual arousal she experienced. However, the women who never did go totally naked also never really relaxed properly, and I could feel that they were still a little stiff and rigid. It seems that for the women who did go totally naked, that once I had seen everything, they relaxed totally, this could be because there was nothing left to hide. If they are still keeping part of themselves hidden, there is always an uneasy tension, or underlying fear that I might see something that I'm not supposed to see. Which is perfectly understandable.

9. It seems to me that a concern for most, if not all of the woman, is that I as the therapist I am trying to get some sexual experience out of the massage. This seems to remain the case for a lot of those who don't go totally naked. However, those who do go totally naked realise in time that this is not the case, and that seems to be part of the healing process. For all the women who finally realise that it is not about sex, there seems to be a mind shift from one where nudity = sex, to one where nudity = trust, nurturing, de-stressing, and happiness. I believe that it is at this point that some women experience an emotional release. This can be a process over time, or a dramatic

emotional release, with tears.

10. It seems that this massage can surface some emotional issues. It confirms the theory that touch can trigger memories of feelings, and memories of hurt. Sometimes just the feeling, and sometimes a memory of the incident that cause that feeling.

In the initial stages it seems that women have to work through these feeling, whether they are negative or positive. If they are sexual feelings, then that might cause them to feel awkward. So they have to get used to that and learn how to respond appropriately. Once they learn that they don't have to act on those feelings, then they start to relax. If those feelings are associated with physical or sexual abuse in the past, then it can be quite traumatic. However, it seems that if they stick at it and continue with the massage treatment, that with time there is a re-framing that takes place, when they realise that nudity and physical touch and massage don't need to be sexual.

For some women, that initial awkward uncomfortable stage can last a few minutes, for others it is a slow process of working though the psychological effects of past experiences.

For some women it's just the awkwardness of having (what they think is an ugly) body exposed, but once they get though that, they relax.

12. For those who are brave enough to go totally naked, the process is not so tricky. For those who are not brave enough to go totally naked, the whole process becomes very tricky. Mostly because they are not going to tell me during the massage that they are not coping. They'll put on a brave face, fake being comfortable, and even make a second appointment, but may not come for that second appointment, because they are too uncomfortable.

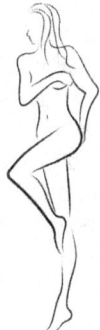

Chapter 9

Why are many women uncomfortable with massage and touch?

This is a question that I have spend a lot of time thinking over. I have considered much of the reading I have done, and taken into account experiences with patients over the years, and I have a number of theories as to why many women are uncomfortable with massage.

Why are many women uncomfortable with massage and touch?

1. The obvious one is that they are uncomfortable with their own bodies, which is the reason for this massage treatment in the first place.
2. Sex/sexuality. Reading between the lines or what some women are saying, they associate massage and touch and nudity with sex, the expectation of sex, or it triggers memories of bad sexual experiences or abuse.
3. Lack of information. If the extent of the massage is more than what a patient is expecting, i.e. They are naked and it is a full body massage, it includes breasts, bum stomach, chest, inner thigh, etc. places that the may be uncomfortable even touching themselves, or seeing in the mirror.
4. Expected levels of confidentiality. Also reading between the lines, some women are scared that I will tell others about them, make fun of them with others, divulge personal, intimate details of their bodies etc.
5. Sexual arousal. It may be that some are taken by surprised, don't know how to deal with their own physical response, and become self concious and uncomfortable with the massage because of it. Time and more massages help to normalise this.

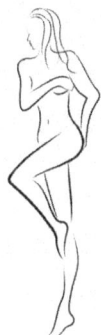

Chapter 10

Theories on what leads to the massage being successful

Again, I have spent some time thinking over this question, and taking a lot of the reading I have done, along with feedback from patients over the years, I have a number of theories as to why massage is so effective.

1. Once the patient has experience the pleasure that can be experienced in their body, the brain makes a positive mind body connection.
2. When they become comfortable with the massage and it is not sexual. Fears can be overcome.

3. Physical touch can trigger memories, fears, and feelings. These can be dealt with in counselling. This would be particularly true in cases of physical or sexual abuse.
4. The physical stress release, can trigger an emotional release. This may also need to be dealt with in counselling.

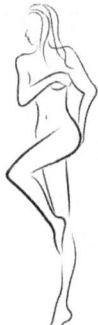

Chapter 11

Real life stories

The question is, how does all this theory work in practice? I'll share two examples from my practice. These are the true stories of two women who have come to me for massage therapy:

Case 1.

In the first example, a female patient of mine who started coming for massages at the beginning of one year, had only been for one back massage. Following that she read that a full body naked massage can be very emotionally healing. She booked a full body massage with me. Nothing significant happened during or after that session, but after the second session, when she was more relaxed about the whole process, she experienced a significant level of emotional release, to the point that when she got home, she burst into tears. She phoned me and asked if it was normal. I have seen this a number of times, so I assured her that it was normal. During her next visit, she shared with me some of her hurts, including leaving home and getting married as soon as she left school, so that she could escape her step father who was emotionally abusive. This patient is a Christian and involved in her church, so after talking further with her, she decided on a course of action which involved going to her pastor for counselling. She has since talked with her mother who apologised for her role, and my patient was able to forgive her mother. Yes, there is a lot of healing still to happen, but the process has been started.

Case 2.

One young lady who has been a client of mine for about five years decided to volunteer for this research. She usually only comes for a back massage. The research encouraged a series of full body massages. Although this young lady in her late 20's has the body of a super-model, she has a body image that is quite different. During her second full body massage, she told me about the allergic reaction she always has to mosquito bites. Because of this reaction she experiences, her mother used to put Jensen Violet on the bites when she was a child. She told me that when she went to school she ended up sitting alone, because the other girls saw all those blisters covered in purple and assumed that she had some kind of infectious disease. This resulted in a poor self-image, and even periods of anorexia. A massage triggered those memories for her, and as she told the story she said "I still react to mosquito bites, but it doesn't bother me anymore". This may seem like an insignificant story, but this is a young lady opening up to me about the hurts in her life, and starting to be able to face them.

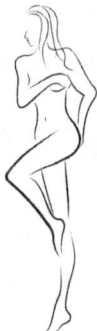

Conclusion

Now that we know how fantastic massage is in improving body image, what do we do with all this information?

Well, there are a number of implications, and applications:

Firstly, for married people, one thing I would like to suggest is that couples take time to massage each other. This needs to be time taken that is separate from sex. Of course sex can follow, but this really needs to be a time when a husband takes time to nurture his wife, and a wife takes time to nurture her husband. Take the time often to give each other a full body massage. Learn to do this properly. Go and take lessons on how to give a massage. You don't need to learn how to be a massage therapist, but just how to give a good massage. The classical Swedish massage is probably the best place to start. It is not a difficult thing to learn. It does require time though.

Giving a full body massage to somebody means that you take about an hour to focus on that one person. If you think that you can't afford to give an hour of your time regularly for you husband or wife, to focus on that one person alone, then I would say that your marriage is already in trouble. What is required is that you need an hour free of distractions. This might mean waiting until your children are put to bed if you have small children. Or it may mean leaving your children with somebody for a couple of hours, so that you can give each other focused time.

An additional option, but not an alternative, is to regularly book massages with a professional massage therapist. I say an additional option, because this should be be done in addition to massaging each other, and not in place of massaging each other, or you will be missing an opportunity to be growing closer to your spouse, and continually developing a close connection.

Secondly, for single people. I would suggest that you book yourself a regular full body massage with a professional massage therapist.

Thirdly, for counsellors, psycho-therapists, psychologists etc. This is a vital tool in the therapeutic care of people suffering with body image problems. Patients should be referred to a professional massage therapist for a regular full body massage. However, it is advisable for the counsellee to start with just a back massage at first. Then over time to progress to a full body massage. Then as time goes on to progress to a massage such as the Hawaiian style Lomi Lomi massage or something similar, which includes full body length strokes. I would suggest that counselling sessions should be booked soon after each massage session in order to debrief the counsellee. Explore the physical feelings, memories, and emotions that might have been unearthed, or triggered during the massage session. It would help greatly if the counsellor and massage therapist are in good communication with each other as well.

Lastly, for healthy people. People who have no physical or emotional or psychological problems. Get a regular massage, just because it is good for you, and keeps you healthy.

"The most powerful thing we can do to help someone change is to offer them a rich taste of God's incredible goodness in the New Covenant. He looks at us with eyes of delight, with eyes that see goodness beneath the mess, with a heart that beats wildly with excitement over who we are and who we will become. And sometimes he exposes what we are convinced would make him turn away in disgust in order to amuse us with his grace. That's connecting. When we connect like that, it can change people's lives" (Crabb 1997:10).

Conclusion

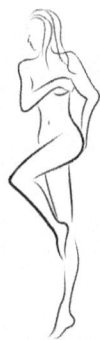

Bibliography

Aneis, D. 2014. *Being Natural: Naked Yoga and it's Psychological Benefits.* In Positive Health Therapy 26 February 2014. (Online) Accessed 24 April 2014.

http://www.dreampositive.info/psychological-benefits-naked-yoga/

Calvert, R.N. 2002. *The History of Massage. An Illustrated Survey From Around The World.* Rochester, Vermont, USA: Healing Arts Press.

Chapman, G. 2007. *The Five Love Languages: How to Express Heartfelt Commitment to Your Mate.* Nashville, TN, USA: LifeWay Christian Resources.

Childline. 2010. *Recognising Child Abuse.* Durban. KZN. South Africa. (online) Accessed 2014-05-08
http://www.childlinesa.org.za/index.php/documents-for-download/doc_download/197-recognising-childabuse

Bibliography

Cowen, V.S. 2011. *Therapeutic Massage And Body Work For Autism Spectrum Disorders*. London, UK: Jessica Kingsley Publishers.

Cosmetic Web. *A Brief History of MTA's Involvement in the Profession*. (Online) Accessed 27 April 2014. http://www.cosmeticweb.co.za/pebble.asp?relid=681

Crabb, L.1997. *Connecting*. Nashville, Tennessee, USA: Word Publishing.

Craffert, P.F. 1999. *Illness and Healing in the Biblical World: Perspectives on Health Care*. Menlo Park, Pretoria, RSA: Biblia Publishers.

Department of Health. 2008. *National Patient's Rights Charter. Booklet 3*. Pretoria, RSA: Health Professions Council of South Africa. (PDF version).

Fletcher, B. 2009. *A Bridge between the Mind and Body: The Effects of Massage on Boby Image State*. Bridgewater, Massachusetts, USA: Bridgewater State University. (online) Accessed 10 May 2014. http://vc.bridgew.edu/cgi/viewcontent.cgi_article=1121&context=undergrad_rev

Fredrickson, R. 1992. *Repressed Memories: A Journey to Recovery from Sexual Abuse*. New York, NY, USA: FIRESIDE.

Fritz, S. 2010. *Mosby's Massage Therapy Review*. St. Louis, Missouri, USA: Mosby, Inc.

Government of the Republic of South Africa. *Regulation published under Government Notice No. R. 127 of 12/2/2001* to be read with the *Allied Health Professions Act. 63 of 1982*.

Hippocrates, in *Peri Arthron Vol. 4 of 10*. Littré (ed) 1839-61, Pairs, France. (Online) Accessed 16 April 2014. https://archive.org/stream/apracticaltreat01grahgoog/apracticaltreat01 grahgoog_djvu.txt

Holey, E.A. Cook, E.M. 2011. *Evidence-based Therapeutic Massage: A Practical Guide for Therapists (Physiotherapy Essentials). Third Edition.* London, UK: Churchill Livingstone Elsevier.

Holland, P. *et al.* 2011. *Chair Massage.* St. Louis, Missouri: Mosby Elsevier.

Kerrigan, C. 2010. *Telling ED NO!: And Other Practical Tools To Conquer Your Eating Disorder And Find Freedom.* Bloomington, Indiana, USA: AuthorHouse

Knaster. *About Mirka.* (Online) Accessed 27 April 2014 Http://www.mirkaknaster.com/index.htm.

Lee, P.J. 1987. *Against the Protestant Gnostics.* New York, NY, USA: Oxford University Press.

Massage Therapy Association of South Africa. *Scope of Practice.* (Online) Accessed 12 April 2014 http://mtasa.co.za/about-mta/scope-of-practice/

Massage School Notes, *History of Sports massage.* 27 February 2014. (Online) Accessed 16 April 2014. http://www.massageschoolnotes.com/history-of-sports-massage/

Maxfield, L. and Dr. Holland, F. 2012. *Client-centred massage has a positive effect on body image: A case study.* Eastleigh, UK: Ferderation of Holistic Therapists. (online) Accessed 10 May 2014.

Mind. Dissociative Disorders. (Online). Accessed 19 May 2014. http://www.mind.org.uk/information-support/types-of-mental-healthhttp://www.fht.org.uk/rr/complementary/massagebodyimageh-problems/dissociative-disorders/#.U3nic4bChMU

Psychology Dictionary. (online) Accessed 10 May 2014. http://psychologydictionary.org/reframing/

Sinclair, M. 2005. *Pediatric massage therapy* (Second Edition). Baltimore, Maryland. USA: Lippincott Williams & Wilkins.

Bibliography

Sinha, A.G. 2001. *Principles and Practices of Therapeutic Massage.* New Delhi, India: Jaypee Brothers Medical Publishers.

Strong, J. 2011. *Strong's Concordance.* Franklin, TN, USA: e-Sword (Electronic Resource).

United States Department of Labor, Bureau of Labor Statistics. *Occupational Outlook Handbook.* (Online) Accessed 12 April 2014. http://www.bls.gov/ooh/healthcare/massage-therapists.htm